Surviving Widowhood

with *Maggie Montclair* and *Friends*

Surviving Widowhood

with **Maggie Montclair**
and **Friends**

PICK A daisy press

Omaha, Nebraska

For information, address the publisher at Pick a Daisy Press, LLC.

Pick a Daisy Press
c/o Concierge Marketing Inc.
13518 L. Street
Omaha, NE 68137

ISBN: 978-0-9849305-1-7
LCCN: 2011962459

AskMaggieMontclair.com

Printed in the U.S.A.
10 9 8 7 6 5 4 3 2 1

csdell

Contents

Meet Maggie Montclair

$\mathcal{T}$he dictionary defines widow as a woman whose husband has died. Widowhood, then, is the living you do afterward. And this book is about how you live the rest of your life.

You will make many decisions that determine just how much joy you find in your remaining years. Even not making a decision is making a choice.

Some of your many choices will be where to live, how to buy a car, whether you will work full-time or part-time or just enjoy being retired. Some will be choices that you can weigh and decide what you would actually enjoy doing. Others will need to be made out of necessity. For example, you may be in a financial situation that requires you to work.

These are just basic everyday decisions. Most of you have experience in these areas, but if your husband handled the checkbook, then you must play catch-up with a good financial advisor.

The important thing is that you do move on— that you do enjoy life again. As you work through your pain, you will realize that grief is not like the flu. You don't get over it. You learn to live with it and not let it rule or ruin your future. Eventually, you will understand how others have survived, and you will again know the joy of living.

Perhaps someone suggested you attend grieving classes. Basically you will share with other women who are suffering the same loss. It helps to know that you are not alone, and the social support encourages you to heal as you see others recovering.

I remember my first class. I was feeling very sorry for myself as I drove to the church basement. My husband had needed a quadruple bypass and a mitral valve replacement. That sounded terrifying, but the doctor said, "Don't worry. He'll leave here in ten days with a smile on his face."

Not quite. Eight days later, he died.

One woman in the class shared her story. She and her husband had decided to go on a Mexican cruise to celebrate their twenty-fifth wedding anniversary. Their two teenagers were staying with grandparents, so they left without a care in the world.

Just before dinner on the third night, her husband had a heart attack. A helicopter flew to the ship and took them to the nearest town with a hospital. No one spoke English.

Her husband lay on a gurney in the hall for six hours. No one would even take his blood pressure. She thought maybe they were afraid to treat him for fear of a lawsuit. She never did find out why he was ignored.

She frantically tried to get them to do something. They ignored her pleas and kept saying they didn't speak English. She just stood by his side and held his hand until he died. When it was obvious that he had finally died, they had his body sent to the local mortuary.

She was able to make herself understood enough to use a phone and call her parents. She planned to bring his body back the next day. She called the American Embassy and learned it could take up to three weeks to get permission to take a body out of Mexico.

She called her parents again (this was before cell phones), and together they decided to have him cremated and bring back his ashes. That would only take a week. Her father was able to fly to Mexico to assist with the arrangements. This was a great help because the "locals" dealt much better with men. They weren't used to working with women, especially a hysterical woman who couldn't speak Spanish.

A week later, she was allowed to bring back his ashes in a plastic bag in her suitcase. By the time she got home, she was in shock. They had his funeral, but her children were still in denial because they hadn't seen his body. Obviously, she had much more to face than her own grief. It would be a long time before her family had joy back in their lives.

When I left that first meeting, I had stopped feeling so sorry for myself. Hearing what others had gone through helped each of us bond and begin our own healing.

I knew that I needed support and encouragement from someone who had survived this great loss and was now happy again. I went searching for a book. There were none to be found. It is my hope that this little book will give you the help you are looking for and make you realize that you have a lot of living left to do.

The important thing is that you do enjoy life again. That you do contribute to society. That your loss does not end your life too. Some of you may be widowed young, as I was, at age forty-nine, or you may have been one of the lucky ones and lived to celebrate your fiftieth anniversary or even longer.

However long you were married, the pain and loss is devastating. Time and support will make the quality of each day better than the day before. Don't give up. Stay in prayer. Remembering to be thankful for all that you have is the best remedy for the "oh pity me" syndrome.

After a month, give yourself just fifteen minutes each day to grieve. You can cry, scream, or beat the walls—whatever you need to do to express your anger, frustration, or sadness.

I gave myself fifteen minutes at noon because that is when I was alone. I was so lonesome that I spent that time crying and feeling sorry for myself. When the timer went off at 12:15, I dried my tears and wouldn't let myself dwell on my loneliness until noon the next day.

One day, I realized that I had forgotten to set the timer. I was healing.

The work of building a new life for yourself is an ongoing process. Do what needs to be done, but add some fun. Do something for yourself that you have always wanted to do. I went to night school for the next two and a half years and finished my college degree. I had to force myself to concentrate and study. I was still lonely, but I didn't have time to sit around and wallow in self-pity.

On these pages, I speak to the most common problems that you will encounter. When you have gone as far as you can on your own, you are invited to join me, Maggie Montclair, in our conversation online at www.AskMaggieMontclair.com.

❀ ❀ ❀

Teaching Grace

It seemed easy, years ago,

To tell the children about the source and benefits of prayer, urging them to converse with God silently, in whatever thoughts were true.

The trick, of course, is open dialog all day, for only five prayers are worth saying anyway:

We praise Thee

We thank Thee

Forgive us

Help us

Into Thy hands …

And if the last is truly sent, to whatever kind of God we can accept, there is no need for other songs. My thanks are already on record, but shall we say a grace today?

To teach the children?

Lois G. Harvey

❀ ❀ ❀

1

Grieving Is Personal

W hen your spouse is ill and you know the end is coming, you wait. Sometimes death is slow and long. Days, weeks, months, and even years go by. Your life is on hold.

Every day you try to find something hopeful. Some sign that the situation is better than yesterday. Less pain. Recognition. New and better medication. When the angels come, you can't believe it is over. Your grief is mixed with relief, and for that you feel guilty. No one tells you that this is the normal reaction, and you are not a monster.

Sometimes death seems to jump up out of nowhere and grab your spouse before you even realize what happened. When you are notified, it is already over. How do you pick up the pieces and put things in order when you are not even able to imagine such a thing?

You hear someone screaming and finally realize that the noise is coming from you. You know you have to get control, so you put your feelings on hold. If you let yourself cry, you will become hysterical. So you hold it in. Just get through the funeral. Just let everyone talk and go home. Just get some sleep, and when you wake up, everything will be normal again.

But it is not normal again. Everything has changed. Now it is up to you to make a new normal for yourself.

You must go through the grieving process and make some decisions all by yourself with no spouse to share the process. Others can suggest, but the final decision is yours alone.

Grieving has been described as a sick feeling in the pit of your stomach, a lump in your throat, an overflowing of tears that just won't stop, insomnia, inability to concentrate, hunger for sweets or chocolate, no appetite at all, chest pains, and headache. There are as many symptoms as there are individuals.

One woman I know gained twenty pounds because she couldn't get to sleep without eating a pan of brownies at bedtime. This is excessive and not recommended, but better than the new widow who over-indulges in too much wine every night. This is a much larger problem than people realize. So beware.

Another widow lost forty pounds and put herself in great peril because she couldn't eat anything. Remember, even in your grief you must use common sense. If family and friends comment on your behavior, pay attention. They have your best interest at heart.

If they say they are worried because you won't go out or see people, you need to have a talk with yourself. Be your own cheerleader and get to a grieving class. They are offered through your funeral home, church, or community college. Working through grief is a tough job and requires help from family and friends.

Usually people with a strong faith in God are able to work through this maze much faster. Change has hit you squarely in the face. The quality of this new life is your own responsibility. If you are waiting for someone else to make you happy, it will never happen. Yes, you are alone. In many ways. This is just one of them. Do what you need to do to survive.

The special advantage of grieving classes is that you meet people who are suffering the same loss.

That shared experience gives you a bond that can lead to new friends. After classes have concluded, many groups meet monthly for lunch. If that isn't suggested, bring it up. Then you'll have a monthly luncheon to look forward to.

Out of that group, a few of you may find that you would enjoy each other's company for other social events. Now, two very important pieces of advice. First, grieving classes are meant to be a "life raft" not a "houseboat." Second, be sure that your new friends have become recovery friends and not always-grieving friends.

Let me share with you some of the letters I received from widows and my responses. I think you'll find some comfort here.

❀ ❀ ❀

Family Man

A quiet man with sudden sparks of wit,
he was fun and funny in his youth,
a Beaver Cleaver little brother who,
when least expected, knew just what to do
to bring a lift. A Mr. Fix-it man
with Can-do grit, good at math and art,
good with plants and animals and babies.

Cogently intelligent, but without guile,
he valued work and went that extra mile
to do things right. His generosity
and honesty were sometimes stumbling blocks,
but always, centered strength flowed out to others.

He became the Patriarch unknowingly.
Worn down by life, missing his own keen edge, he
yet found humor in indignities
of illness—called laughing attention to
his last, enforced Tim Conway shuffle.

A steady love, not overspoken,
rock safe and sure in good times and in bad,
a family man who took his roles seriously,
but never himself: True Heart, Brave Soldier,
Lover, Husband, Father, Grandpa, Friend.

Lois G Harvey

❀ ❀ ❀

Dear Maggie Montclair,

I know you are not supposed to make big decisions for at least a year, but this house reminds me of Don to the extent that I'm depressed just being in my own home. Everywhere I look I see reminders that he is gone, and I break down from missing him.

Once when I was fixing lunch, I even thought I heard him calling to me from the living room. I can't move right now or afford all new furniture.

Is this normal or am I losing my mind? What can I do?

Gone But Not Forgotten

Dear Gone,

Some women find it necessary to remove all his clothing and personal belongings. Some get by with removing just a few items. Some save everything for a while because it gives them comfort.

Each of us grieves and receives comfort in our own way. Go through the items in your home and get rid of those that cause you pain. How about his favorite chair? If it just sits there, making you miss him even more, get rid of it. You might want to offer these items to your children. What gives you pain may comfort them. You won't know unless you ask.

When you have purged your home to your satisfaction, then purchase something new for each room. It doesn't need to be expensive: a plant, stove burner covers, throw pillows, different colored towels, sheets, a small rug. Make at least one change in every room.

Some women find that adding several feminine touches to the bedroom makes a huge difference. A new bedspread, or something pink with ruffles—anything that defines the room as a woman's bedroom. Keep adding items until each room feels like you, not him.

And, no, you are not the first widow to think she heard her husband calling to her. Our mind plays tricks on us to remind us just how fragile we are. If you are not already in a grieving group, now is the time. $\mathcal{M}$

P.S.: My dear friend Gertie has a cousin whose best friend's sister was widowed ten years ago. She hasn't moved a thing since he died.

His newspaper is still on his recliner! No one has sat in his chair or touched the now-yellowed and crumbling paper. His half-empty coffee cup is on the table beside said recliner. The coffee has long since hardened and separated from the sides of the

BEST DAD mug. His clothes are still in his dresser and hanging in their closet.

Everything is ready for him to magically reappear and continue living. Only immediate family have been in this house since that fateful day. And she only goes out when absolutely necessary.

This "shrine" is witness to the fact that two people died that day, but only one was buried. ✿

Dear Maggie Montelair,

People say, "Call me if there is anything I can do for you." Is it all right to say they can help me by just going out to lunch with me? And that I need someone to visit with and be normal with? I know that sounds pathetic, but that's the way I feel right now.

Pathetic in Georgia

Dear Georgia,

You're on my mind. And the minds of others. People offer their help in this way for a couple of reasons. If they haven't been widowed, they really don't have a clue about what you need right now, and they do want to help. They are often afraid to suggest an outing for fear it is too early, and you will turn them down. Sometimes, they just don't think something so small as a lunch date will be helpful.

So, the next time that happens, just say, "Thank you. I would really like to go to lunch with you. What day are you free next week?"

Set a date and show up with a smile. Have a "normal" lunch. No tears or pity-pot stuff. This will help you stay in touch with your friends.

In fact, you don't need to wait for them to offer help, just call and invite someone to lunch. M

P.S.: My wonderful friend Gertie's next-door neighbor's third cousin's hairdresser was widowed three years ago. Sadly, she has lost most of her friends and many clients because she is the queen of pity and doom. She takes every opportunity to share her sadness and tears. No matter how good a day you are having, she can bring it down. Everyone wants to run, not walk, to get away from her.

Her widowed clients tried to talk with her and explain that she needed grieving classes so that she could feel better. Her response was that no one, not even other widows, could possibly understand her sorrow. She said that her marriage was so much better than theirs and her grief so much stronger that she will never be able to get over it.

Unfortunately, there are too many widows who don't want to go to the work of building a new life. Gertie told me, "She thinks people are saying how sad for her that she loved her husband so much that the rest of her life will be spent mourning him, when actually people are thinking that she has 'gone round the bend,' so they keep their distance." ❀

Dear Maggie Montclair,

I survived the time in the hospital and the funeral by telling myself that I just had to hold on and get through just one more task, and then everything would get back to normal.

Finally, I've written the last thank you note, returned the last dish, and sorted and given away most of his things. Now, tell me. How much longer before my life is normal again?

Waiting in Montana

Dear Waiting,

Everyone has a different normal. Your normal was with your husband. Now, you have to make a new normal for yourself under very stressful conditions.

This is the time to reflect on the best part of your past. Make a list of all the wonderful things you did together in your old normal.

Now, go over that list and see what you can put on a new normal list that you can enjoy by yourself or with a friend. For instance, if you and your husband enjoyed the theater together, you can still get joy from that activity, but you will either need to go alone or with a friend.

Maybe you enjoyed all the ball games that your grandchildren played. Your new normal can still have those games to enjoy. Keep enjoying life for the both of you.

Your new normal can include things that you always wanted to do. Maybe you always wanted to try your hand at painting, but didn't want to leave your husband alone while you attended classes. Now you can sign up for those lessons and enjoy yourself. Maybe your secret ambition has been photography or to write a novel. Go for it.

Make your new normal as exciting as possible. Chances are, you will meet new friends who will enhance your life even more. $\mathcal{M}$

P.S.: Gertie's painting instructor's next-door neighbor was widowed at eighty. She is one of those rare people who loved being with teenagers. She had enjoyed her own children and her grandchildren. She decided that she wanted to do something where she could be with kids again. But how?

What could she do? Then, as luck would have it, she stopped in at her local McDonald's for a cup of coffee and noticed a HELP WANTED sign. She filled out the application and interviewed with the manager. By the time she finished her coffee, she had the job.

Two weeks later, she collected a paycheck. The first one in her life! She spent the next five years working at McDonald's as one of their most valued employees. Who knows how many teenagers she helped.

When she retired, every former employee who still lived in the area came to her party. They hugged her and gave her cards of appreciation. She is one happy woman! ❀

❀ ❀ ❀

A friend told me that about three weeks after the funeral for her husband, her daughter and grandson came to visit. The little guy bounded in and snuggled up to her on the couch. He looked up at her and asked, "Where is Grandpa?"

Her daughter said, "Now, Gabe, remember we talked about Grandpa going to heaven?"

Without missing a beat, he said, "Yeah, but, Grandma, did he take your car?"

She and her daughter enjoyed a much-needed laugh.

❀ ❀ ❀

❀ ❀ ❀

Do you not ask me how I am

for fear of causing me pain?

Do you not shed a tear

for fear of causing me to weep?

Do you not ask me about him

for fear of causing painful memories?

I understand your fears

I have had them, too.

Yet, now that I am the one hurting

I know it's not questions, tears,

or memories that hurt.

It is your silence.

Nicole E. Hildreth

❀ ❀ ❀

Dear Maggie Montclair,

It has been a year, and I just can't move on. I've been to classes at the funeral home, grieving classes at my church, and coping classes through the community college. Nothing tastes good and I have to force myself to eat. I am tired all the time because I don't sleep at night. My daughter says this will pass, but I'm tired of feeling so bad.

When will I wake up and feel happy?

Trying to Smell the Roses in Nebraska

Dear Sweet Rose,

Remember, grieving and coping classes are meant to be a life raft, not a houseboat.

One class, if it is a good one, will be all you need. All the hard work must be done by you. Talk positively to yourself. Be your own cheerleader. Talk yourself into having lunch with friends, going to movies, and inviting people to your home. Go to your church functions, take a continuing education class in art or photography. Whatever interests you. Find a place where you feel comfortable and volunteer. It really is hard work building a new life.

That still doesn't mean that you will feel bubbly every single day. It still doesn't mean that you will never have another sad day. It just means that you are putting some joy into your life. The more you make positive choices, the easier it becomes. The more you do things with and for others, the less time you will spend thinking about your loss.

You are making a whole new life for yourself. You are learning to live as "one" instead of being half of a couple. Of course, it's hard.

You may think that others are moving faster than you, but part of recovery is personality, part is family support, and the biggest part is hard work that can only be done by you.

If you have done as much as you can and are still sad most of the time, talk to your doctor and share your situation. You may be suffering from depression and need medication for a while. Never be embarrassed to get the help you need for a good life. You are in charge. Do what it takes to be happy. $\mathcal{M}$

P.S.: Gertie's favorite bank teller's sister's neighbor was having health problems when her husband died. This compounded her grief and recovery. She just couldn't quit crying. Her daughter took her to the doctor who prescribed an antidepressant. She refused to take it because she considered it a sign of weakness.

The poor lady spent another six months in misery before her daughter was finally able to convince her that this wasn't something that was due to a lack of strength or intelligence but a problem that was both physical and emotional.

Why do we, as women, expect to go through everything by ourselves on sheer willpower? Maybe it is because we have always been the strong ones who took care of everyone else, and it is hard for us to admit there is something that we can't do by ourselves, just because it needs to be done. We get to be stubborn old women who won't let anyone or anything help us.

For our own good and those who love us, we have to get past this attitude. ❀

Dear Maggie Montclair,

I know this must sound terrible, but I smiled all the way home from the cemetery. So did my three children. Free at last! He was foul-mouthed, physically abusive, a tightwad (with his money and mine, I had to sign my paycheck over to him), and a demanding father.

My children have never brought up his name, and neither have I. It is as if he never existed. He was what my parents used to call "a street angel and house devil."

Ironically, they had one in their own family and never knew it. They loved him! If I had tried to divorce him, he would have gotten all the support, and my children and I would have been seen as making mountains out of mole hills.

What do I say when other widows talk about how much they miss their husbands? So far I have kept quiet because no one would believe me anyway. All of our friends, and everyone in town thought he was a loving family man.

Giddy in Galveston

Dear Giddy,

You have been wise to keep your private life private. The old saying, "Never speak ill of the dead," is still around for a reason. If you "speak ill" you are saying more about yourself than you are about the dead. And it is not a flattering statement.

Just because a man is dead does not mean that he was a good husband, father, or even a good human being. It just means he is dead. If no one misses him, he did not live well. And it's all over for him, anyway. At least here on earth.

When you are in a group, you do not need to respond. Just listen. If you are required to make a response to a direct question, you can truthfully say that it is a challenge to begin again or any true statement that mimics the group feelings. You can agree that they miss their husbands without making the statement for yourself.

Just remember to be gracious. It will be in your best interest. Some things need never be confided. This is one of those things. The sooner you move on with your life, the better. You may want to skip the grieving class and go straight to more social activity with other widows. $\mathcal{M}$

P.S.: When Gertie's mother's bridge partner's husband died, she drove everyone crazy talking about what an "obnoxious excuse for a man he was." She listed his faults and had a three-minute speech that she loved to repeat to anyone who would listen. It got to the point where everyone tried to avoid her.

The gossip among us girls was that maybe he wasn't so great, but living with her would drive anyone to drink. She didn't get the sympathy she craved. Instead, she got criticism. ✿

2

Lonely—or Alone?

To be alone is often a choice. To be lonely is a suffering of circumstance. Loneliness is a deep hunger for companionship that demands action on your part. Because it requires a proactive response, you might often find it easier to continue with this known miserable state than to risk the unknown by trying to change the situation.

So you have two choices. You can continue the status quo and complain that you are lonely, or you can make a list of activities that will give you pleasure and an opportunity to make new friends. With list in hand, do what has to be done to find those new friends.

Your list might include these activities (and I'm sure you'll think of many others):

- Go to church and get involved in activities and groups there.

- Go to a senior center.

- Join a walking club (through the Y or your neighborhood community center or employer).

- Join a weight loss group (if you need it).

- Take lessons: swimming, dancing, bridge, computer.

- Volunteer at the hospital, elementary school, or nursing home.

- Get a part-time job if you're not currently working.

- Join a widows' group (if you can't find one, put an ad in the newspaper or search local blogs or start one).

- Join a Red Hat chapter (those ladies know how to have fun). If yours is dull, be queen of a new chapter.

If you are working full-time, you will need to check your local paper for evening and weekend activities that will let you meet new people. If this were easy, there wouldn't be any lonely people. So do something that makes you feel good: get your hair done—and your nails and get a pedicure—then say a prayer, put a smile on your face, and go meet some new people. Forget about yourself and be interested in them. There is a whole village, town, or city full of interesting people that you will enjoy knowing. Go find them!

I am often asked about how to fight loneliness. Here are some of the letters from brave ladies who wrote to me. I invite you to email your questions to me online at www.AskMaggieMontclair.com, especially if you don't find just the precise answers you are seeking here.

Dear Maggie Montclair,

I have been a widow for almost three years, and I still dread eating alone. Sometimes, after eating over the kitchen sink, I'm not even sure what I just ate! Something out of the fridge. Something quick. I know I'm not eating healthy. What can I do?

Eating My Heart Out

Dear Lonely Heart,

This is one of the main complaints of every widow. You are not alone. Not by a long shot. So be inventive. Try different plans. Good china. Sit in the dining room.

If that's not your cup of tea, how about eating in front of the television? I know experts say that is a bad idea, but unless they are widows or widowers and can tell you a way to enjoy eating alone, I'm not sure their plan will be any better than what you come up with.

Probably the best way to enjoy a meal is to share it. Invite someone over or meet a friend at a restaurant. You don't need expensive, you just need company. Make a list of all the widows you know and start calling. Set up three or four lunch dates. Your current meals won't seem so bad when you have those to look forward to.

If you do come up with the perfect solution, be sure to share it. Many widows would certainly be grateful for your secret plan on "eating single." *M*

P. S.: My friend Gertie eats out as often as possible. She claims, "I've never met a meal I didn't like." When she has to eat alone, she fills her plate in the kitchen and then quickly puts everything away. She enjoys her meal in front of the TV, and if she wants more, she has to mess up the kitchen to get it. She finds this usually keeps her from overeating out of loneliness or boredom. ✿

Dear Maggie Montclair,

I am so lonely. My friends are all married. I have season tickets to the symphony, but they either go with their husbands or won't leave their husbands to go out for an evening. And then some of my friends don't enjoy the symphony. It is a fifty-mile trip to the city, and I don't want to drive alone, even if that was an option.

This is a fairly small town with no grief classes, so I don't have a way to meet other widows. I'm shy by nature, so starting something would really be a problem for me.

Lonely in Rural Michigan

Dear Country Girl,

Let's do some critical thinking. First and foremost, you are lonely. What are your options? You can do nothing and remain lonely, or you can go against what you consider your "nature" and take action.

Call the funeral home and ask if they would consider starting a grieving class. If they say yes, you can offer to help them with the first meeting by taking cookies or something.

If they say no, you can put an ad in your local newspaper stating that there will be a "Dutch treat" luncheon for all the widows in town at such and such a restaurant at noon on Wednesday. Let the restaurant know what you have done. Even though you have absolutely no idea how many women will show up, it is courteous to alert the restaurant.

As the women arrive, greet them and give them a name tag. You will be wearing one, of course. All you have to do is give a short welcome and then go around the table and have each attendee introduce herself. Visit with each other and plan to meet again next week. You can make lists of everyone's name and phone number and email address to pass out next week.

If no one shows up, you can eat alone or go home. Either way, it is not the end of the world. As word gets around, you will probably have a larger crowd every week. Get to know these women and invite a few that you want to know better to your home for lunch.

This group can get as large and active as it decides. Now you have several women who might want to share your symphony tickets and other life experiences. I know many women who enjoy bus trips together. When ten women get together, it's a party! $\mathcal{M}$

P.S.: My friend Gertie loves people. It's her "nature." One evening she was clearing off her desk and computer station. She found a 1-800 number scribbled on the edge of a newspaper. For the life of her, she couldn't remember why she had written that number down or who it belonged to. So she called. Turns out, it was a late-night radio talk show. The topic for the evening was "what stress does to you."

Gertie jumped right in, and the talk show host loved her. He was especially thrilled with her because she was well into her "senior" years, yet her mind and spirit were young and vibrant.

Gertie said it must have been a slow night because they talked for over ten minutes. Now, they talk every month on the show. If Gertie is busy and doesn't call by the middle of the month, he calls her. He told her that his listening audience loves their conversations.

The reason I'm telling you about Gertie is to suggest that if your "nature" doesn't give you enough fun, then push yourself a little. Get out of your comfort zone. Don't use your "nature" as an excuse to live a lonely life. ❀

Dear Maggie Montclair,

When my husband died, I was left to grieve and care for our mentally challenged son who had grown into adulthood. His father was able to keep him under control and handle his temper tantrums. It became more and more difficult for me to keep him calm. When I became afraid of him, I knew that I had to make a change.

After many inquiries, I was able to find a group home that would give him a chance. That worked for a short time. Changing his meds and moving to another group home has been the story of our lives for the past five years, but it still is better than living in fear. I hope he will calm down as he ages.

I am now able to take some trips with a friend and go to a widows' group. I am busy and thankful for group homes and the staff that does their best with difficult patients.

I hope that sharing my experience will help others realize that sometimes the choices are hard, but necessary.

Made the Tough Decision in Texas

Dear Tough Lady,

You really were between a rock and a hard place. You are a strong lady to do what is best for both of you even when it breaks your heart not to be able to mother your son.

God bless you both. $\mathcal{M}$ ❀

Dear Maggie Montclair,

My children are insisting that I move. I have lived in our home for fifty-six years and have no intention of leaving. My son took care of my lawn and snow removal until two years ago when he injured his back. His son took over but is now going to college out of town and interning during the summer.

We are having a problem getting dependable help, but I am willing to put up with that in order to stay here. They worry about my health and being lonely. I tell them to leave me alone and let me do what I want.

Don't I have the right to decide where I live?

I Want to Stay Home

Dear Stay-at-Home,

Your children love you and worry about you. Humor them a little and don't be so cranky.

Have plenty of food in case you get snowed in. Have flashlights for power outages. Do whatever you can to make yourself safe.

Maybe you will be one of the lucky ones and die peacefully in your sleep. Pray that you aren't one who falls and gets hurt and can't get help right away. Or one who gets sick and can't reach anyone. At the very least, wear a help button around your neck.

You could hire an agency to have someone be with you a few hours each morning to help with your shower and light housekeeping. They will take you to doctor appointments and to get your hair fixed. They take you to the grocery store or do the shopping for you. There are many good agencies out there. They screen the women they send to help you, and many become good friends. If they cook you breakfast and lunch, your evening meal can be something out of the refrigerator.

Maybe taking these actions will satisfy your children. *M*

P.S.: Gertie's brother's mother-in-law's sister wouldn't move from her home even though it wasn't safe for her to be alone. Her eyesight was failing. She failed her driver's test and lost her license (and the kids took the car). She wouldn't hear of hiring anyone to come in to help her or even use a health alarm. She was one of those I'll-do-it-myself people.

Well, she really did it herself! She fell and broke her hip during a snowstorm and power outage. It was three days before her children could reach her. She had been dead for two days. Was she conscious?

Did she suffer? No one knows. Her children said she had plenty of money but just wouldn't spend any on herself. She was that way all her life and she died that way.

Gertie smiles when she tells about her friend who went kicking and screaming to an assisted living residence. She was determined not to be happy about "what her kids did to her." But after a few days she couldn't resist playing BINGO. She also discovered that there was a group of pinochle players looking for another player. So, of course, she had to check them out. Then there was the singing group that needed an alto. She had loved singing in the church choir, so she joined them. The Red Hat Ladies were always laughing and going out to restaurants for lunch, so she donned a red hat and went with.

Within a month, her calendar was so full of fun that she told Gertie, "I should have come here two years ago." ❁

Dear Maggie Montclair,

My thirty-year-old daughter is mentally challenged. When my husband died six years ago, I thought Sue and I would be able to live together and even enjoy many activities. However, that was not to be.

Her hormones went out of control, and I couldn't even take her shopping without her yelling inappropriate things to men in the mall. She even tried to touch them. They could immediately see that she was not a "normal" woman and quickly moved away.

When she began sneaking out of the house in the middle of the night, I added birth control pills to her daily meds. However, that couldn't keep her safe from the people she might meet out on the street. When I had to pick her up from the police station, I knew her life was in danger if I didn't make some changes.

After she repeatedly ran away from the group home where I placed her, they wouldn't take responsibility for her safety. My last recourse was to make her a ward of the state where they keep her in a secured environment.

Sadly, she is not happy being there. I'm beside myself with guilt. I just don't know what else I could have done. I can't even think about going out and having fun when my daughter is so miserable.

Guilt Ridden in Reno

Dear Devoted Mom,

How sad for both of you. Every mother wants her children to be happy, but no matter how hard we try, it is not always in our grasp.

Please find a counselor that you like and can share all your feelings with. You may have to visit with more than one therapist before you find one you click with. Over time, you will come to realize that you had to take this drastic step to keep your daughter safe.

Those of us on the outside can see that this was your only option, and we realize how difficult it is for you. The important thing is that you realize this and don't feel guilty for protecting your daughter. A good therapist will get you to this point. Then you will be ready to live the rest of your life with joy. $\mathcal{M}$ ❀

Dear Maggie Montclair,

I have been widowed for almost a year. And I have an embarrassing problem. I am afraid to be alone at night. I hardly sleep and then nap or am tired during the day. I don't want to take sleeping pills.

I told my children that I didn't like being alone at night, so they installed an alarm system. They don't want me to sell the house because it is the family home, and they have all their "growing up" memories here.

I shared my fear with a widow friend who moved to an independent living community right after her husband died. She told everyone that since she didn't have any children living in the area, she didn't want to bother with finding people to take care of her property. She confided to me that the real reason she moved was because of fear.

I want to live where she lives. She doesn't have to eat alone. A bus takes her on trips and to the theater. She still has her car and is free to do as she wants, but most important of all, she is never alone at night.

I want to tell my children that I am old enough to do what I want and if they love this house so much, they can buy it from me. What do you think?

Terrified of the Dark

Dear Sunshine,

Show this letter to your children and admit that you wrote it. They probably have no idea how afraid you are. They want what is best for you, and your current situation is obviously not working out. It is not good for your mental or physical health to be so frightened and sleep deprived.

You know where you want to be and what you want to do. When they realize that you have a place picked out, they will understand that this is going to happen, and they will help you. That is what loving children do for their parents. Maybe one of your children will want to purchase your home. At the very least, they can each take items of importance to them—their growing up memories—after you take what you want for your new apartment.

Liking a new place is 90 percent attitude, and you have that mastered. Enjoy your new home. God bless. $\mathcal{M}$

P.S.: My friend Gertie's neighbor's favorite aunt's husband's second cousin was also afraid to live alone. She made her house into an actual fortress. With all the special locks, alarm systems, and screws in the window slides, she was still terrified.

Her children dragged her to a psychologist who asked her what would make her feel safe.

She thought for a while and decided that nothing anyone could do would make her feel secure. If her children weren't willing to live with her, she wanted to live in a retirement home. She could play cards and visit with others whenever she wanted. She could watch her favorite television show and share popcorn. She could just sit quietly and crochet.

The unanimous decision was that she was more lonely than afraid. She desperately missed the presence of her husband and that manifested itself as fear. She is now happily crocheting a winter scarf for every resident of her new home. ❀

3
Friends and Acquaintances

$\mathcal{H}$ow did life get so complicated? We go through the trauma of losing our husbands and then find that we have to search for new friends.

What happened to those married friends we have known for years?

Suddenly, they are just too busy. Or they act as if they think we are trying to steal their husbands. Maybe they think widowhood is catching, and they haven't been vaccinated. That leaves us alone when we are most vulnerable. If you already have widowed friends, you are lucky. If you are the first in your group, you have some work ahead of you.

Some friends "jump ship" at the first sign of tragedy, just as others desert at the first sign of good fortune such as a new man in your life. You can't change the actions or reactions of others. Just realize that their actions say more about them than about you. You must forgive those "busy" friends. For whatever reason, they don't realize how much they are hurting you. If they become widows, welcome them with open arms. They will need you.

You can be assured that I get plenty of letters from widows asking me about these so-called fair weather friends. You're not alone. Here is what I tell them.

Dear Maggie Montclair,

I have been widowed almost a year. I have joined a widows' group that has many social activities, and I go to most of them. I am pleasant and nice to everyone, but it seems there is some unspoken rule that I don't know about. I can't think of anything that I could have done to offend anyone. I have even entertained some of the women at my home. But they're just not warming up to me.

Should I just give up and try to find another group or should I keep going and hope that the women will eventually accept me? I'm so lonely for friends.

Suzanna from Savannah

Dear Suz,

Sadly, your situation is much too common. It seems as if many women in these groups act as if they were back in junior high. Without their husbands, they become insecure and cliquish.

If you move to another group, you may well find the same problem. Tough it out. Befriend new members as they come into the group. Be kind to everyone—even those who are not friendly—and do not get caught up in gossip. Give everyone the benefit of the doubt.

If you are not enjoying this group after a year, then by all means find another group. This is why so many groups fade away. When ladies are not made to feel welcome, they don't come back, and the group dissolves. Good luck. $\mathcal{M}$

P.S.: My friend Gertie has a way of looking at bad behavior. She figures the people are either in pain that day or they are suffering from a lack of oxygen to the brain. Both of these situations can make a person cranky. If they are always cranky, it is probably the oxygen problem, and they most likely won't be around too much longer.

Either way, don't take it personally. Some women just have to know everything about everything and always be in charge. It is what it is. ❀

Dear Maggie Montclair,

I have been widowed for three months and still feel terrible. Yesterday, one of our friends called and asked me to lunch to talk.

However, it was not the wife (I'll call her Marie) who called. It was her husband, Ed. I have known this couple for thirty years and never felt he was attracted to me. But the thought of lunch alone with him makes me uncomfortable. When I suggested that Marie come with us, he said that would be fine another time, but he thought it would be good for me to talk with just him.

Somehow, that doesn't make sense to me. I finally agreed to meet him next week, but I'm having second thoughts. Is this a perfectly innocent lunch, or am I reading into it things that don't exist? What do you think?

Questioning in Quincy

Dear Questioning,

It is never a good idea to meet a married man alone for lunch or any other time. Why would you want to risk a problem? Rumors start even when something is totally innocent, and a simple lunch gets turned into something ugly. There really is no free lunch.

Ask him to have Marie call you when it is convenient for both of them to meet you for lunch.

I heard a radio minister talk about avoiding the sharp corners in life. This is one sharp corner, sister. And I'd avoid it. Just say no. *M* ❀

Dear Maggie Montclair,

It has been two years since Joe died, and I am having trouble making new friends. We had several friends who are couples, but I didn't have any single friends.

The couples have been wonderful to me and include me in dinners and the theater, just like before. They don't seem uncomfortable, but I am. I'm always the fifth, or the seventh wheel. I let them bring another man along a time or two, and that was even worse.

I'm not interested in a man. At least not now. What do you suggest?

Driving Me Crazy in Wheeling

To You in the Driver's Seat,

It sounds as if you are ready to move on and enjoy the rest of your life. This will require some effort on your part.

Visit some senior centers. Keep looking until you find one that meets your needs and has widows around your age. Some give art lessons, have card groups, singing groups, exercise groups, book clubs and more. Become a part of what interests you and look for widows you would enjoy seeing outside the center. Center hours are during the daytime, so you don't have to worry about being out late at night.

Check out the Red Hat Society at www. RedHatSociety.com. You will find a list of chapters near you. These gals plan fun activities, travel together, and really know how to laugh. If you want to go on a cruise or travel to Europe, this is your group. Safety in numbers! No one messes with a gaggle of happy women wearing large red hats! They just stop you to have their picture taken with you.

The library offers book clubs and opportunities to volunteer your time to read to children. Volunteering not only helps others but gives you a chance to be with other age groups. Good for the soul.

Don't forget your church. They have women's study groups and committees. Many have singles groups. They always welcome newcomers, and you will be doing something for others. The happiest women seem to be those who make time to help other people.

Some towns have "Widows Clubs." They meet for dinner, go to movies and plays, and rendezvous at each other's' homes. Join a group or start one.

Go have some fun. $\mathcal{M}$

P.S.: My friend Gertie attracts friends like most people attract mosquitoes on a hot summer night. Wherever she goes, she meets the most interesting people, and somehow they become friends. She says her theory is the same as that television channel that says "characters welcome." She doesn't judge, criticize, or advise. She just enjoys listening to their stories and then shares a condensed, humorous version of her own. (She has buried four husbands, and that in itself is quite a story. No, she didn't murder any of them.) ❀

❀ ❀ ❀

Arlene of the Pink Moon

Arlene, the waitress at the Pink Moon
Diner out on Route 69 is a celebrity.
For more than a year now she has not cut
(nor broken) the two middle fingernails on
her left hand. Folded into her palm for
protection, they have grown into four-inch
curving crimson-coated claws. Truck
drivers have quit noticing her blond curls
and pert breasts. Instead, they inquire
about her fingernails: "Anything broke
yet, Arlene?" Highway travelers glance
sideways as she carries cups pinched
between thumb and forefinger, the prized
showpieces extended.
Two more inches should get her on TV.

Lois G. Harvey

❀ ❀ ❀

Dear Maggie Montclair,

What is wrong with me? Why are my former friends ignoring me? Last week while getting groceries, a friend since grade school stopped me in the canned vegetable aisle and said, "I was in your neighborhood last week and thought about you. It's so good to see you."

If she was in the neighborhood, why didn't she stop? She used to stop for coffee at least once a week. Should I call her and ask her what is wrong?

Something Wrong in Colorado

Dear Colorado,

By all means, go ahead and call her. But instead of asking her what is wrong, ask her to meet you for lunch. Or a movie. Or both. No tears. No, "I'm so lonely." I know it is asking a lot of you, but you need to be the one to put her at ease. She couldn't tell you what is wrong even if she tried. How can she put into words that she doesn't know what to say to you? She doesn't want to make you cry. She doesn't want to say the wrong thing, so it is easier to just stay away.

It is a common situation, and you may still lose many of your old friends, but you can at least make the first move to keep those relationships intact. It really is worth the effort. ℳ

P.S.: Gertie's first husband's cousin's barber's brother had the opposite problem. When his wife died, he described the ensuing onslaught as "an army of single women with covered dishes." He even had to start keeping a calendar of his dinner invitations. Within the first year, he had three marriage proposals. He has managed to stay single for two years now, but even he says, "My resolve is weakening." ❀

4

Family Togetherness

----

 f you are lucky, you have family that will support you through your grief. They can't do the work for you, but they can assure you that you are loved and cared for. Just knowing that helps you more than they realize.

Most of us put on a strong front for our children, regardless of their age. We know they are already suffering to their limit with the loss of their father, and we don't want to add to their burden. If you're like me, you hold it in.

Some of us are lucky and have a sister or friend (like my friend Gertie) whom we can call at 2 a.m. when we are falling apart. They are our special angels. We shouldn't expect our family to take over and do everything for us for the rest of our lives. We have to learn how to go on living—and they know that too. We do hope we will be included in their family parties and continue to share in their lives. Our grandchildren become more special than ever.

We hope our sons-in-law and daughters-in-law will understand that we need to have our children extra close for a while. Death seems so near, and it scares us. This passes as we get our bearings and begin to heal. Our family needs to help us decide the best place for us to live. These days, there are so many options.

Many of us, depending on our age and finances, stay in our own homes. Some enjoy senior apartments, others want a regular apartment, and still others want assisted living.

If you are leaving a house where you have lived for many years, it can be a strain on everyone concerned. If cost is a factor, your choices will be limited. Don't forget that you can live anywhere and get help through private agencies or state and federal agencies when you need it. Don't pay for services that you don't need yet. Don't act "old" before you have to.

We all want to keep our precious driver's license as long as possible. While you are still driving, offer rides to others. Carpooling is fun and saves gas. There does come a time when it is best to stop driving. Your children aren't being mean, they are trying to protect you. After all, it means more work for them!

Pay friends well for taking you with them to activities and shopping. With the cost of gas, they will probably thank you for the contribution and your company. Always be on time and willing to adjust to their schedule.

And drivers, at night and even in the daytime if no one else is around, please wait until your passenger has entered her home or building. I remember reading about a son who dropped his mother off and drove away. She fell on her steps and froze to death.

His fate was worse than hers because he spent the rest of his life regretting his actions. If he could just do it over, he would walk his mother to the door, unlock it for her, and turn on the lights. He would give her a hug and a kiss. He would wait outside until he heard her turn the lock. She gave him life; he could at least have protected hers in this simple way.

Gertie's brother's wife's best friend knows a woman with several children who started a wonderful, loving tradition after their father died. One, two, or more of the kids would stop for coffee on their way to work. Just for a few minutes to make sure their mother was up and dressed and ready to start her day.

They don't realize what this did for her. In the beginning, it forced her to get out of bed, even on those days when she wanted to stay under the warm covers and not face reality. Even when her heart was breaking from loneliness. But she left her memories on her pillow and made the coffee.

Now, years later, they still come. They can connect and share, not only with their mother, but with each other. What better way to start a day?

Here are some of the letters I have received on this topic.

✿ ✿ ✿

Memo to Myself

Go ahead

keep your loneliness, wrap it around you

like a cloak.

Climb your battlements

to gaze beyond.

missing joy

here at your feet.

But remember, he who builds walls

leaves fences unmended ...

Lois G. Harvey

✿ ✿ ✿

Dear Maggie Montclair,

I have a wonderful, well-educated, beautiful daughter. She has a prestigious job and is well known throughout the metro area. One of her business associates told her that she saw me with my Red Hat friends and we looked like we were really having a good time. This embarrassed my daughter because she thinks I should refrain from public gatherings with what she calls, "Hatted old ladies."

I told her that the point of the group was to go out to play and have a good time. We do have fun, but we aren't disruptive or loud. People do come up to us and want their picture taken with us, and we are always polite and friendly.

I told her that I was sorry if I embarrassed her, but I was not going to change my behavior just because she was so stuffy. Now she is mad at me. We haven't spoken in a week, but I'm sure it will blow over.

It's really kind of funny. Like she is the mother and I'm the teenager.

Do I need to act old and stay home by the fire?

Having Too Much Fun in Fargo

Dear Fun-Luvin' Gal,

As long as you are always a lady, go have fun. When you are in a restaurant, you know how to behave so you won't be disruptive. Just make sure that you never have to call your daughter for bail money. $\mathcal{M}$

P.S.: Gertie is the queen of fun. Whenever her phone rings after 10 p.m., she knows it is her neighbor the dairy "Queen" with a late-night craving for ice cream begging for company on her late-night jaunt. Gertie slips her old garden jeans over her pj's (prays she isn't in a car accident) and is out front in five minutes ready for a hot-fudge-sundae run. When she did this at seventeen, she never dreamed she'd be enjoying the same adventure again at age seventy-eight. Go have fun.

All the laughing makes it worth the effort. ❀

Dear Maggie Montclair,

I have been widowed for three years and thought everything was going as well as could be expected and even better in some areas of my life. Now, I find that I need serious surgery.

I am terrified, but I don't want to tell my children how scared I really am because they are already panicked. I know that if I share my feelings with my closest friend, she will think she needs to tell my children. I want to grab a stranger off the street and tell them that I'm not ready to die yet. Or even worse, be incapacitated and be a burden to my family.

Scared to Death in Ohio

Dear Scared to Death,

I'm so glad you shared your fear with me. I know it is not like having someone give you a big, warm hug and tell you that everything will be okay. But I am doing just that in my heart.

What I can suggest is that you write a letter to your children and share your love for them along with all these feelings. My guess is that when you get it all on paper, you won't be as scared. Prayer is helpful to most of us. People seem to find that praying for strength to face the future and giving thanks for all the good that is in their lives gives them a calmer perspective.

When you have written everything you want to say, hide the letter in your house. When you are well again, you can decide whether to destroy it or share it. Your children won't ever know about the letter unless they are sorting through everything in the event that you don't recover. $\mathcal{M}$

P.S.: Gertie's great aunt's neighbor left a letter for each of her children. She updated the letters every New Year's Day. She told them how much she loved them and how happy she was to be their mother. She praised their accomplishments and told them how proud she was of them and their children. She specified which of her belongings she wanted to bequeath to them. The next day, she took each new letter to the mortuary and added it to last year's envelope. She used that time to update or change her funeral plans. By the time she needed the services of the mortuary, she and the funeral director were old friends. ❁

Dear Maggie Montclair,

I just turned seventy-four, and, believe it or not, I'm still raising children—my grandchildren.

I have the precious darlings ten hours a day. I love them dearly, and they are my pride and joy. At first, taking care of them made me feel young and brought back the fun memories of raising my own children, without the sleepless nights. I thought this was the perfect world.

But now, after a recent knee replacement, I find that I am exhausted by the end of the day. Last week, I stumbled while carrying the baby and almost fell. I keep thinking about what could have happened if I hadn't been able to catch myself. It is probably not safe for the children, but what would I do all day? Do I dare risk their safety? Advice, please.

Worrying Grandma

Dear Grams,

How would we ever forgive ourselves if one of our precious grandchildren was hurt on our watch? Most people don't realize just how much strength and muscle tone is lost after age sixty-five until they get there themselves. Or how exhausted we get.

It sounds like your child care days should be over. Look around at your friends. Once they enter their seventies, the aging process seems to accelerate. Heart problems begin. Bones become fragile. Diabetes rears its ugly head. Balance is compromised.

This is not the time to be responsible for young lives. It is the time for your last hurrah! Have fun with your friends. Take every opportunity to enjoy your day. Don't end up in a nursing home wishing you had "gone out to play" with your friends.

You are responsible for your own life, not your daughter's life, and your own level of happiness. If you weren't around (and I mean like in Florida for the winter, let's say), what would your daughter do for day care? She'll figure it out.

You have spent your life taking care of a husband, children, and probably a job. Now it's time to take care of yourself. Do it well! *M*

Dear Maggie Montclair,

I have been widowed for four years and am doing quite well. My health is exceptionally good for my age, and I have many fun friends.

However, my son is worried about my safety. Granted, the neighborhood has gone down hill these past few years. He thinks that I should buy a gun and take lessons to learn how to use it. I have never liked guns and think maybe a Taser would be better. My daughter says I would probably end up shooting myself or the mailman. She thinks that because I will be seventy-eight next fall that I should move to a retirement apartment.

I'm really wondering what would make me the safest. Do you have any suggestions?

Trying to Be Safe in Kansas

Dear Trying to Be Safe,

I think your daughter has the right idea. A gun or Taser might be the answer for someone who has had a lifetime of experience with guns. But to start with weapons later in life can be quite tricky and not the best idea for most of us. Even an experienced person needs to give careful thought to the fact that her eyesight and steadiness may be impaired.

But let's look at the bigger issue here: Your safety. It is hard to relocate. Check with your friends who live in retirement buildings and see how they like living there. If you moved where you already know someone, it would make the transition much easier. Many of my friends say how much they appreciate the fact that during a storm, they are not alone. If the power goes out, they get together with flashlights, junk food, and cards and have a party. Then safety is not a serious issue for them. $\mathcal{M}$

P.S.: My friend Gertie's dentist's son's best friend was working as a landscaper during summer break between his junior and senior year in college. He happened to see a stray dog running down the middle of the street, and being a nice, caring young man, he scooped up the pup and discovered on the collar that the cute little guy lived about three blocks away. His boss gave him permission to return the dog, so he carried him to the house, went up the steps, and rang the doorbell. That's when the trouble began.

The lady of the house came to the door with a can of wasp repellent, saw a dirty, sweaty kid with her precious doggie in his arms and taking no chances, pushed the nozzle. The spray went right through the screen, saturating both the good samaritan and the dog. Later, she explained to the officer, "I heard you should shoot first and ask questions later." ❀

Dear Maggie Montclair,

My friends and I were having lunch last week when the subject of those alert buttons you wear around your neck or wrist came up.

One woman said her doctor said that anyone over fifty who lived alone should have one just in case of a fall or illness.

A few of the women in the group had them and told us how much safer they felt—both for health and safety reasons. If someone is breaking into your home, you can use it to call for help. They are not expensive for the security they afford.

But the main reason I'm writing is because one woman said she could be dead in her house for days before one of her children would find her. They call when they need something, and they leave a message if she doesn't answer. She is really on her own. We were surprised how many in the group had the same experience.

Why is this so common? Our children don't hesitate to ask for favors or money, but they never call just to make sure we are all right or to ask if we need help with anything.

Help, I've Fallen …

Dear Fallen,

I don't know why some children seem to be more concerned for their mother and father than others. Maybe it is hard for our kids to face the fact that their parents are getting older and may not be as strong as they want them to be.

Most children do love and appreciate their parents. It seems they lead such busy lives with work and their own children. Their inattention is usually not deliberate, just an oversight. Forgive them. You raised them and maybe you didn't teach them to show appreciation for gifts and acts of kindness and they have an "I deserve" attitude.

Or maybe that was just one of your lessons that they ignored. Whatever the reason, refusing to run to their aid or write that check may give them a wake-up call. We all need to feel loved and cared for without begging for attention. *M*

P.S.: My friend Gertie's former college roommate has an amazing daughter. The kind every mother hopes for. She lives over a thousand miles away, has a husband, three young children, and a job. Yet she calls her mother every morning at 7:30. Her husband and children have just left for work and school when she pours herself a cup of coffee and has a ten-minute chat with her mother before she heads for work. She finds out her mom's plans for the day, doctor appointments, or results. She makes sure her mother sounds strong and is up and beginning her day.

Jane loves these quick calls. She finds out what the family is doing, how school is going for the children, and knows her daughter is well. On Saturday she talks with the grandchildren and her son-in-law. They don't see each other as often as they would like, but they certainly keep in touch, and Jane feels loved. ❀

Dear Maggie Montclair,

It used to be so much fun to spend time with my grandchildren. I take each of them out to lunch and shopping. They choose the restaurant and the clothes they want for school or summer vacation. I have always looked forward to this special time with each of them.

Now, two of them are teenagers, and it is not much fun for me. They spend their time texting instead of visiting with me. One even talked me into taking her best friend with us. They left me in the dust except when it was time to produce a credit card. I even ended up buying an outfit for the friend!

I can't believe that my grandchildren have become so rude and greedy. What can I do?

I Don't Like My Grandchildren

Dear I Don't Like My Grandchildren,

Unfortunately, your situation is much too common. You can be a grandmother who loves those teenagers enough to teach them manners that will help them through the rest of their lives. Think back. How would your grandmother have reacted to such inappropriate behavior?

This is the age of technology, and in some ways, we need to adjust. But manners are as important today as when we were learning them. It is our duty to be sure that our grandchildren know how to treat us. We do that by telling them.

When it is time to go shopping, make the plans as usual. Then say, sweetly, of course, "I don't want you to bring your phone or friends with you."

If they complain and threaten not to go, just say, "I'm so sorry that you don't want to go. I love you so much and I'll miss not having that time with just you. But, my dime, my rules. Call me if you change your mind."

When you put the ball in their court, they learn to think things through and weigh consequences. $\mathcal{M}$

P.S.: Gertie's manicurist's cousin tried this with her college-bound granddaughter. This girl was really full of herself and told her grandma that if she couldn't take her phone, Grandma could just keep her dime! Grandma did. At Christmas when the older and wiser young lady came home for the holidays, she told Grandma that she was ready to go shopping without her phone. Grandma gave her a hug and said, "Oh, honey, I spent that dime on extra Christmas gifts for the family. I'll save up and we can go shopping when you get home for summer vacation." Believe me, this grandmother now has six grandchildren who treat her with respect. ✿

Dear Maggie Montclair,

I just got home from the funeral of a dear friend. It was so sad and upsetting to see her children arguing with each other. One of her sons was upset because my friend had been cremated. I know this was her wish, and her other children respected that request and outvoted him. But I think this has permanently ruined the relationship among the siblings.

I have a daughter who is always at odds with her brothers. How can I be assured that my funeral won't cause similar problems?

Don't Want to Buried in Michigan

Dear Don't Want to Be Buried,

The loss of a parent is so stressful that unresolved anger toward a parent or siblings often surfaces. If the relationship is already tenuous, these feelings can cause a rift that may last for years. There are a few things you can do to help avoid this situation.

You can go to the mortuary of your choice and make all of your own arrangements. Even pay in advance. This will take pressure off your children at a time when they are most stressed. They won't have to decide how much to spend on a casket or if you would want to be cremated (often a problem), what music you would want, or if you preferred flowers or memorials to a charity. Your mortuary will have all these questions, and more, for you to think about and decide.

When your decisions are made and everything is paid for, ask for copies of the entire contract and decisions you have made and send a copy to each of your children. Tell them that if they have a problem with any of your decisions, they are to call you directly and not discuss it among themselves. If you don't want to make any changes, then everything will be as you planned. $\mathcal{M}$

P.S.: Gertie's next-door neighbor's mother's best friend went one step further. She thought her children were rather stuffy (she always said that she couldn't figure out how that personality trait found its way into her gene pool) so she even planned the viewing. She had purchased an urn that looked kind of like a large sugar bowl with a curvy lid. It was to be placed next to her picture (it had been taken when she was about fifty) on a wet bar that would be moved into the mortuary and provide free champagne for everyone. The background music would be Frank Sinatra singing, "I Did It My Way."

By the time this all took place, she was ninety-six years old. Unfortunately, all her friends had already passed and were not there to enjoy the festivities. But her great grandchildren thought she was one nifty nana. ✿

Dear Maggie Montclair,

I have been widowed for four years and was doing quite well until last year when my sister's husband died. She sold her home and moved in with me. We have always gotten along well, and I thought we would enjoy each other's company and both save money.

She brought so much furniture and boxes of "stuff" with her that I should have been suspicious, but I just moved my things to a corner and let her fill up the basement. Later, I noticed that she was bringing packages from all the stores in the shopping center but not showing me her purchases.

When I went to the spare bedroom for some extra towels, there were all the sacks with the items still in them. The room was so full that I couldn't get to the closet. I went to her room to ask her about her shopping sprees, and when she opened the door, I could see that her room was so full that she could hardly get to her bed. In fact, the bed was piled so high with clothes, she had a sliver of room left in the bed to sleep.

I was too shocked to say anything at that moment. I was trying to figure out how to broach the subject when the next day we ordered pizza, and she wouldn't let me put the empty box in the trash. She said it was

*too good to throw away and that she would take it to
her room and use it for storage.*

*When I told her that I didn't want her to do that
because it might draw bugs, she got angry, grabbed
the box, and stormed to her room.*

*Maggie, what can I do? I've seen those hoarder
shows on television, and I can't live like that. But I
just can't throw my sister out either.*

Smothering in My Own House

Dear Smothering,

You have to address this situation right now.
Before it gets any worse. And it will. Hoarding
is a mental illness that requires specialized help.
Does your sister have children? If so, contact them
immediately and tell them you have an emergency
situation that they will have to deal with. Explain it
to them and then take action to protect your home
and sanity.

Explain to your sister that the two of you can
no longer live together. Tell her that she has a
hoarding problem, and even though you love
her with all your heart, you are not capable of
helping her with this. Take her to check out some
apartments and insist that she sign a lease. Call a

moving company and have all her items moved to her new apartment.

Locate a therapist who specializes in treating patients with hoarding disorders and offer to make her an appointment and go with her. She probably won't be willing, but you have planted the idea and can write the doctor's name and number on a large piece of paper and stick it to the kitchen wall above her refrigerator. If she ever changes her mind, she will have the information.

Have her visit you from now on and treat her with love and affection. Remind yourself that, through no fault of her own, she has a serious illness. You can be a loving sister without allowing her to destroy your home and sanity. $\mathcal{M}$

P.S.: My brave friend Gertie has personal experience with hoarding. She loves to tell about the time when she was a child of six and went with the neighbor girl to visit her grandmother. Grandma's house was a maze of bundled, stacked newspapers. Gertie was immediately lost and became hysterical. An adult found her and lifted her into the air so she could see where she was in relation to the door. Needless to say, Gertie never went visiting with her friend again. In fact, she claims to be afraid of newspapers to this day unless they are accompanied by a cup of coffee. ❀

Dear Maggie Montclair,

I guess I don't really have a problem. Just a question.

My daughters and daughter-in-law are busy, modern young women with important jobs. Their husbands take on much of the household responsibilities and child care—much more than the men of my generation ever dreamed of doing. They use throw-away plastic forks and paper plates. They don't keep their clothes (something about style) or their cars as long as my generation did. Their pictures are all in their digital cameras and most don't even get printed.

I'm just wondering, what can I leave them and my grandchildren that was a part of my life that they will want to keep as a way to remember me? My good china that I saved for over two years to purchase? I don't think so. Maybe my wedding silver? No, too much work keeping it shiny. How about my grandmother's favorite potato salad bowl? Do they want anything from my past? Is that even important to this young generation?

Barking Up the Wrong Family Tree

Dear Solid Oak Mama,

Many young people are interested in their roots. The genealogy websites attest to this. How about leaving them a written account of your life along with your personal items? The items will mean more to them if they realize how much they meant to you.

You can tell the family stories that have been passed to you, tell them about your parents, grandparents, and even great grandparents if you were lucky enough to know them. At the very least, you can tell them what you knew or heard about those people. You can enjoy the memories as you write them and only tell the flattering things about yourself. How fun is that?

If you really want to give stuff away, include the family potato salad recipe with the special bowl, and give it to one of your granddaughters at her wedding shower. Family recipes are a legacy to treasure and pass on. $\mathcal{M}$

P.S.: Gertie's family tree, as you can imagine, has some very twisted branches. She researched her crazy Uncle Herman, the one with the gold mine in California (or so he said) and the spinster aunt who taught school in New York City at P.S. 141. She has written a family history for her descendants and included some family secrets. Her lawyer has a copy of this history, and copies will be given to each of her family members when her will is read. Maybe there's a treasure map for that gold! Personally, I would love to be there and get a copy! ✿

❀ ❀ ❀

Remembrance

What will you keep of me?

One line? One flower?

One hour?

That which a lifetime cannot tell

Can death bestow?

What you will keep of me

I do not know, I do not know.

Lois G. Harvey

❀ ❀ ❀

5

A Man:
To Have or to Have Not

Are you interested in another man? Many widows would like to marry again.

Maybe they had such a good marriage that they want a repeat, or maybe theirs wasn't so great, and they want to try again. Many women would like a man as a companion to date and spend quality time with. Or some want a strictly platonic relationship. Others are ready to forgo any relationship with a man and spend their days with family and friends.

If all you want is a "man," that's easy. Just go to any bar at closing and someone will be eager to go home with you.

Most of us don't want that kind of relationship. We want a relationship with a decent man we can proudly introduce to our family and friends. They are out there. The world is full of good men. Just be careful when you are looking. I hope you have friends who can introduce you to someone they know to be honorable. If not, you may want to try Internet dating. Just be careful.

If you connect with someone online, meet him during the day in a public place such as a Starbucks or the museum or a restaurant. Drive yourself, and do not give him your address. Get to know him during daylight hours and continue driving yourself until you are confident that he is trustworthy.

Getting back in the game is tricky. Here's what I have advised some of my new dear friends.

Dear Maggie Montclair,

I have been widowed for three years. For the last two months I have been dating the most wonderful man. We see each other almost every day, and when we can't, he calls several times. We enjoy the same things and laugh all the time. He pays attention to everything I say and always compliments me on my hair and clothes. When I am with him, I feel young again.

The problem is my daughter. She points out what she calls "red flags." It is true that I have not met any of his friends or relatives. I have not been to his home, and I have loaned him a small amount of money that I am sure he will repay when he gets his next dividend check.

Are these so-called red flags really important, or can I tell my daughter to quit worrying and let me be happy?

Fannie in Flagstaff

Dear Fan,

Your daughter is waving some very important red flags.

Ask yourself how much you really know about this new guy. Where did he work? Has he been married before? Does he have children or other relatives in the area? If not, why is he living in your city?

The answers to these questions should have come up in normal conversation. Is he reluctant to talk about himself? Take it slow and get all the answers before you make any promises or lend him more money.

Your daughter can do some Internet searching too. It's amazing what you can find out about a person. And of course you could check into having a private investigator snoop around at Mr. Right's past.

Let your daughter know what you are discovering and let her help you decide if this man is all he claims to be. If she hasn't met him, invite both of them to lunch at a nice restaurant so they can become acquainted. She wants you to be happy and safe. Go slow and be wise. *M*

P.S.: Gertie knew a woman who met the perfect man. She thought he was the man she would love for the rest of her life. It was a whirlwind courtship, and she found herself married before she hardly knew what happened.

It didn't take long to regret her haste. Turns out, he wanted "a nurse and a purse." He recognized her lonely and generous heart and was right there to take advantage.

She called a divorce lawyer and corrected her error in judgment. It cost her some money and pride, but not nearly as much as if she had stayed with him. She told Gertie that even old fools can change their minds and get smart again! ✿

Dear Maggie Montclair,

I have been widowed for almost ten years and have just begun getting Social Security. I have been dating a widower for the past year, and now that we are both sixty-five, he thinks we should each retire and live in my house. He would sell his and pay half the expenses at my house.

I have a couple problems with his idea. First, even though I like him very much, I'm not sure that I want him around 24/7, and I don't want to have to cook three meals a day and do his laundry. I told him that I have lived alone so long that I didn't think he would enjoy my constant company. He promised he would adjust to me.

Second, what if he doesn't follow through and pay his half? The thought of having more money is appealing, but I wonder how long we would agree on what to buy. He says we can solve that by having legal papers drawn up declaring exactly what would be purchased and what he would pay.

But probably my most important concern is our health. I took care of my husband for three years before he died. He was the father of my children, my faithful husband, and the love of my life. I would have continued to take care of him forever.

But John and I don't have that history. If he gets sick, I don't want to take care of him or have him take

*care of me. John refuses to discuss our health saying
that I am looking for problems that don't exist.
How do I resolve this situation?*

Tilly in Tucson

Dear Tilly,

You have already decided that living together is
not the right plan for your future. Don't let him
change your mind. You are in charge of your own
life. Don't do anything unless you are eager to
enjoy a new situation.

Listen to that warning voice. *M*

P.S.: Gertie's second cousin's ex-brother-in-law's
sister got tangled up with a man who had a habit of
marrying widows and spending their money. He
divorced them rather quickly and usually came out
ahead financially. The last she heard, he had just
divorced his fourth widow. He made the comment
that widows were more trusting and therefore
much easier to beguile. We should strive to remain
trusting, but not gullible. ❀

Dear Maggie Montclair,

I have met the most wonderful man, but my friends and family don't like him. They say he is controlling and keeping me from them. That is not true. I really would rather be with him. He pays attention to me and listens to me. He doesn't enjoy being with them because he can feel that they disapprove. I haven't met any of his friends or family. He says he doesn't want to share me with them.

He wants to get married, but I think it is too soon. We've only known each other three months. He says, if I love him, I'll marry him right now and live happily ever after. I do love him, but worry when he says I have to prove it by doing what he wants.

My son is threatening to hire a private detective and have him checked out. What should I do? I don't want to lose him.

I Do But I Don't in Des Moines

Dear Do and Don't,

If you "lose" him because you won't let him dictate your actions, you never really had him. Getting married after a three-month courtship isn't good for anyone at any age.

Every couple needs friends and family. He may be enough for you right now, but that won't last. No one stays in the "honeymoon" phase forever.

When it wears off and your life together begins, you need a strong commitment and respect for each other. Not infatuation. If he won't see your point of view, then let your son check up on him. You might be surprised what you discover. $\mathcal{M}$

P.S.: Gertie's son's best friend's father was a private detective for an insurance company. He said it is amazing what people are hiding. He dug up lots of dirt on both men and women he investigated. He found bigamists, grifters, and even ex-cons who had failed to mention their incarceration to their new love.

Some men (and women) have a lot of baggage. Be careful out there. Look inside the Samsonite. ❀

Dear Maggie Montclair,

My daughter is upset with me because I have started dating a seventy-two-year-old widower. I'm sixty-six. I have been alone for six years, and I thoroughly enjoy our time together. He lives in the next block, so we go for walks, share many meals, and garden together—vegetables at his house and flowers at mine. We think it is great fun.

We will not marry or live together, but just enjoy each other's company. We are planning a bus trip this fall and will have separate hotel rooms.

My daughter knows all of this, but she thinks this is being unfaithful to her daddy. She was always her daddy's little girl, but this is too much. She told me that if I don't stop seeing Tom and cancel our bus trip, she will cut me out of her life and not let me see my grandchildren.

My son-in-law tried to talk some sense into her, but she accused him of taking my side and told him to stay out of it. In order to keep peace at home, he refuses to discuss it with either of us. I just can't give up my grandchildren. But giving in to blackmail really bothers me. I will never again feel the same about my daughter. She has broken my heart.

Your devoted follower,

Milly in Philly

Dearest Milly,

Your daughter has put you in a no-win situation. How sad for all of you. Is there anyone who could talk to her? A clergy person? Even wedding vows say "until death do us part." The Bible gives everyone permission to love again after the loss of a spouse.

If nothing you do will change your daughter's mind, then you have to make a very tough decision. Tell her how she has broken your heart. She is using her children as blackmail to get what she wants. Her father would not be proud of her as one of his best qualities was his understanding of other people's needs, and he loved his family so much that he wouldn't want his wife to be lonely for the rest of her life.

If she still refuses to budge, then you decide if you can live without seeing your grandchildren. Your daughter may miss you enough that she will grow up and realize she can't get what she wants by blackmail.

If blackmailing works on you, God help her poor children. They will never live a life of their own. $\mathcal{M}$

Dear Maggie Montclair,

I want to meet a man to spend time with. I miss talking sports and going to games. I miss the give and take of a relationship, and I want someone to get dressed up for. I am tempted to check out Internet dating.

None of my friends would approve, so I don't have anyone to talk to about it. I mentioned it to my sons who said it isn't safe and to put it out of my mind. What do you think?

Dateless in Dayton

Dear Dateless,

You might be wrong about your friends not approving. Bring it up as a what-if situation. At least a few might be interested and want to discuss the possibility of Internet introductions, not only for you, but for themselves as well. You might be starting something fun for all of you.

There are many good men out there. Maybe you will meet one that you have a lot in common with. Just be smart and meet in a public place until you are very sure of him. Let your sons know what you are doing and where you are going. Good luck. *M*

P.S.: Gertie has a friend who signed up with an expensive dating service because she thought that anyone who could afford this agency wouldn't be looking for money. Maybe they didn't need money, but some rather strange people did sign up.

One date kept his gloves on while he ate his whole meal. She admitted it was a cold February night, but they weren't on a picnic for Pete's sake. They were in a warm restaurant. That was her only date with him.

Then there was the quirky guy who was looking for someone to drive to Maine with him in a U-Haul full of empty plastic water bottles that he had collected to redeem for a nickel each. He figured that would pay for a nice little vacation on the East Coast. She gave him the boot.

Then there was the man who couldn't dance or bowl because he had a steel rod in his back, couldn't go to movies because he was claustrophobic, couldn't eat in restaurants because of food allergies, and didn't play cards. When she asked what he wanted to do on a date, he said, "Have someone come to my house and cook with me and watch television." She ran to the nearest exit! ✿

❀ ❀ ❀

Altergeist

Two years you have been gone

and I bear the loss one day hard, one day soft.

I carry memories

one day close, one day far, wondering where you are.

Your spirit stayed with me;

I opened doors expecting

you to be there, held my

pillow at night as you.

Once I heard your voice

calling so clear that I got up

to see if you were here.

Nightly the phone rang with

no one answering my hello.

Mornings there was tapping

at a window, the source unseen.

Even after the tears stopped

I thought of you day on days.

*Gradually the pain decreased, new busyness filled
my mind, I stored a widow's weeds.*

Yesterday a man held me

in his arms and we danced.

Last night at midnight

when I was alone, the floor

moved like a quake and some

*unseen force lifted the foot of my bed and
let it drop.*

Today I let that man

hold me in his arms again.

*We kissed and it felt right, though different
from you.*

Are you still here somewhere?

Do you know what I ask?

Will you shake the house down

Around my ears if I

Should take him to my bed?

Lois G. Harvey

❀ ❀ ❀

6
Moving On

$\mathcal{M}$oving on is finding your old self again and planning a new life. The changes will be in you and in making new friends.

Meeting new friends may be part of that moving on process. Do you think every person you meet is going to like you? They won't. Don't be disappointed.

Sometimes new friends are too critical. Maybe your smile reminds her of the little girl in third grade who pushed her off the swing. Maybe your laugh grates on her nerves. Maybe she thinks you wear too much make-up or jewelry. Maybe he thinks you are too fat. He is seventy, but he is so handsome that he thinks he should be dating a slim fifty-year-old. Maybe you are too high maintenance when he is looking for a petite woman who loves cooking and cleaning.

Who knows. It doesn't matter. It's none of your business what others think of you. Be friends with those who treat you right and keep your distance from those who don't. But you never have the right to be mean to them or gossip about them. Try to stay far away from that junior high girl that you once were. Remember, some women are seventh graders forever.

Understand that as we age, we get tired much more quickly than in our youth, and many of us get cranky. Some even go beyond grumpy to downright cantankerous. If you are one of those, as I am (I blame it on the need for a nap), it is important to "keep thy mouth shut" and not respond to others, or you will surely be sorry for what you say.

Forgive others for their lapses, and don't let it ruin a friendship. The next lapse may be your own. Remember, your tongue is the only muscle in your body that is attached at only one end! It needs less exercise than other muscles!

Make it a point to see how many wonderful friends you can have before you leave this earth. Meet people with a smile and introduce yourself. I met a ninety-six-year-old "young" woman at a

Red Hat gathering. I asked her the secret for such a long life. She said that her last thought every night before going to sleep is to plan something that she will do for someone else in the morning. What a wonderful way to enter dreamland.

I get so many letters asking about when to move on or what moving on really means. Maybe you'll find some answers for yourself in these responses to my very dear readers. But first a sweet poem:

❀ ❀ ❀

In Memoriam

My brother says

no one is dead

until the last person

who knew him

is also gone.

I read of a man who

had kept a record

since childhood

of every person

he had ever met.

I wish I had done that.

I am sure it would be

more than two thousand.

And I intend to

keep on meeting people.

Lois G. Harvey

❀ ❀ ❀

Dear Maggie Montclair,

My doctor told me to get a treadmill and walk thirty minutes every day. I bought the treadmill, and my son-in-law set it up. That was the easy part. I just can't force myself to go down to the basement every day and get on the darn thing! Help.

Treading on Thin Ice

Dear Ice Skater,

You aren't really lazy, you just put that darn treadmill in the wrong place! Unless your bedroom has more action than mine, no one but you needs to see it. So make that darling son-in-law his favorite pie and ask him to come move it one more time.

Now here's the plan. As soon as your alarm goes off, turn on your bedroom TV, and get on that treadmill for fifteen minutes. Now, with half your exercising done, you can bring in the paper, make scrambled eggs in the microwave, pour a glass of juice, put on the coffee, grab a paper towel and take your breakfast back to bed. If this means a few extra steps, just think of it as needed exercise. Avoid toast unless you enjoy vacuuming sheets.

Directions for an enjoyable breakfast are as follows: arrange pillows to support your back, check the weather, the morning shows and finally the early morning movies. Read your favorite part of the paper and settle in. That little remote is all yours.

You can linger with your coffee, watch television, and read the whole paper before doing another fifteen minutes on the treadmill. Or as soon as breakfast is finished, you can do the treadmill and enjoy your coffee and paper after your shower.

You can accomplish a great deal in a short time and still have the rest of the day to enjoy. If you have never tried breakfast in bed, don't knock it. How many times did you get out of bed to fix breakfast and take care of the family even when you were so sick that you should have been the one receiving care?

It's no one's business where you choose to eat your breakfast, but if this little luxury makes you feel guilty, then just don't tell anyone. You are old enough to have a few secrets! $\mathcal{M}$

P.S.: My friend Gertie has a cousin whose former boss's ex-wife is so committed to breakfast in bed that she has added a small college dorm refrigerator and microwave to her bedroom décor. She told Gertie that there are days when she becomes so captivated with an old movie that she stays put until lunch. Take a lesson from this savvy lady and have breakfast in bed with Tony the Tiger. ✿

Dear Maggie Montclair,

I have adjusted to widowhood and have a happy and full life. There is one thing I would like to do, but it seems a foolish waste of money. I want to take piano lessons.

When I was a child, my parents couldn't afford it. My husband thought it was an extravagance, so our children didn't have the opportunity. Now, my neighbor is moving and has offered to sell me her spinet at a very reasonable price. I can afford both the piano and lessons. I want to begin each day by making music.

The only thing stopping me is wondering what my children and friends will say. I'm wondering if when they ask me why, is it enough to say, "Just because it is something that I've always wanted to do."

Want to Make Music in Maine

Dear Music Maker,

I wonder why so many of us think it is necessary to validate our actions. If you can afford it, and it won't hurt anyone, and it's not immoral, why do we even give a thought to what other people might think?

I read that when people are on their death bed, they regret what they didn't do much more often that what they did do. After I read that, I got the courage I needed to write this little book. If some people don't like it, well, to be honest there is no book that everyone would like.

What might have stopped me would have been if my children would be embarrassed. As it turns out, they are thrilled and totally supportive.

So I think you should give yourself those hours of music. What a wonderful way to start each day! $\mathcal{M}$

P.S.: Gertie has a wonderful outlook on trying new things. She just does whatever she thinks will be fun. She has painted some lovely pictures. She writes poetry. She made a CD of herself singing her favorite Christmas carols (slightly off-key), and she learned to tap dance at age seventy-two. Her only fiasco took place during a cake decorating class. All she will say about the incident is that there was a kind of "frosting explosion," and they asked her not to return. ✿

Dear Maggie Montclair,

I am doing quite well after two years of widowhood.
I am busy doing what I enjoy and have several new
friends. My problem is that we go out to lunch so much
that I have gained much more weight than I should.

I don't want to give up my friends and our lunches,
so what can I do?

Regretful in Gainesville

Dear Regretful,

This is a universal problem among all women
whether they eat out or not. Eat healthier choices
during your lunches (maybe split a meal) and get
some exercise. Have a talk with your doctor.

Weight gain can often be attributed to
medications that we are taking—and maybe not.

Good luck. M

P.S.: Gertie's neighbor's mother-in-law gained
forty pounds the first year that she was widowed.
She panicked at the thought of eating alone, so
she called her friends and went to lunch with a
different friend every single day.

On top of that, she hosted dinner parties every
weekend with family, neighbors, or her church
guild. When she could no longer get into her
clothes or stand to look in the mirror, she knew

she had to make a change. She decided that she just couldn't give up her food dates, so she joined a gym. It took six months at the gym and careful menu choices, but she was able to get her weight under control and still enjoy her social life. She has made even more friends through the gym, so she now has breakfast dates too with the ladies from the water aerobics class. ❀

Dear Maggie Montclair,

I needed a dress for my nephew's wedding. It was to be my first social event after the funeral, and all of my family would be present. I wanted to look especially nice. So I grabbed my credit card and headed for the mall.

The twenty-something clerk gave me "the look" and listened while I told her my situation and explained how important it was that I look elegant. I interpreted "the look" to mean "another old lady wanting something that doesn't even exist."

I simply wanted a dress with sleeves that would cover my bat-wings. A waist that really was on my waist, not below my naval. Long enough to cover my knees, without looking "dutchy."

I ended up paying way too much for a pant suit that I don't really like and probably won't ever wear again. Why won't manufacturers make clothes for the more mature woman? We seniors do have money to spend. And we still want to look nice.

Naked in North Dakota

Dear North Dakota Naked,

Wouldn't it be great if the producers of the old *Golden Girls* television show had a garage sale to get rid of the clothes? Sophia was supposed to be in her eighties, yet she always had stylish clothes, no matter what the occasion. Dorothy had outfits that covered her pop-out tummy that tends to arrive as we age. Rose wore beautiful dresses.

Now, Blanche, well, she was different. She wore all styles and whether we agreed or not, she always thought she looked absolutely stunning. Maybe she had the right idea. Maybe if we think we look gorgeous, others will think so too. Or at least they won't have the nerve to tell us we don't!

As the Baby Boomers age, the manufacturers just might design beautiful clothing for older women because of the "size" of the market. Our job is to live that long. $\mathcal{M}$

P.S.: My friend Gertie, always wanting to be in style, decided to eliminate the dreaded panty line by wearing a thong. She bought the largest one she could find. In black lace.

On the way to dinner she told us that she was fully aware of the fact that it would take some getting used to. But she reminded us she was determined. She squirmed during the salad. She grimaced during the main course. Before dessert arrived, she returned from the ladies room with the thong in her purse and relief on her face. We have noticed that her panty line is back. ✿

Dear Maggie Montclair,

Last week while I was getting my hair done, I glanced in the mirror and saw my mother. I was absolutely shocked!

My old aunt had been telling me for years that I looked like Mom. I just couldn't see it. But since that fateful day in the shop, I have seen my mother in several mirrors.

I loved my mother dearly and really don't mind looking like her. It's just that I have always thought of myself as an independent individual. Now I have to rethink that assumption and realize that we actually are tied to our DNA. I wonder how my daughter will respond someday when she sees me in her mirror. I hope I am still alive!

Mirror, Mirror on the Wall

Dear Fairest One,

Remember that nursery rhyme where the old witch says, "Mirror, mirror on the wall, who's the fairest of them all?" Did you ever look in the mirror and claim, "I'm the fairest of them all?" No one would admit to that. Even on her best day. Even when she was twenty. Even when she was slim.

I once read that men and women see their reflections differently. A woman looks at herself and sees every flaw. Real or imagined. A man, on the other hand, sees his reflection, smiles, and thinks, "Pretty darned good."

My husband, God rest his soul, was a wonderful man. However, on more than one occasion, I observed his mirror smile and wondered just what he was thinking. He was definitely pleased with the view. $\mathcal{M}$

P.S.: My oldest friend Gertie says that when she looks in the mirror, she sees a fat blonde, unless, of course, she's just had another hair coloring accident. She has tried every color while looking for that perfect shade. In reality, there aren't that many hair colors on the planet, but she just laughs and keeps looking.

Whom do you see in the mirror? Tomorrow morning, take a lesson from the men. Smile into that mirror and say, "You're looking pretty darned good!" ❀

Dear Maggie Montclair,

When I worked, I dressed up every day and wore high heels. Now, ten years later, I'm a retired widow and rarely get out of my sweatpants. I recently joined a group of active widows who go out to eat every weekend at upscale restaurants where I could start getting dressed up again.

The problem is that I've gained thirty pounds so none of my out-of-style clothes even fit. I want to lose the thirty pounds, get all new clothes, and wear high heels again. Not the five inch, but nice two and a half inch. Am I dreaming, or can I really look and feel attractive again at seventy?

Feeling Dowdy in Florida

Dear Feeling Dowdy,

Go for it! There is no reason why a seventy-year-old cannot be an attractive, vibrant, charming woman. Actually, age has nothing to do with it. Most is attitude. The rest is determination to be as healthy as possible and to spend time on packaging. M

P.S.: Gertie plays bridge with a woman in her early nineties. She couldn't believe this beautiful, intelligent woman's age. She eats healthy, has her hair done in an attractive style, wears a little make-up, and dresses in well-put-together outfits. She looks expensive and elegant, but in reality is careful to choose clothing that is flattering to her slim figure and coloring. She has overcome cancer, a broken hip, and various other ailments. Her biggest attribute is her attitude. Always a smile. Always upbeat. A joy to be around.

Gertie decided to emulate this lovely lady by getting rid of her glasses and getting contacts. Her optometrist recommended that she stay with glasses and update her frames. But you know Gertie, she insisted on contacts.

We never knew anyone could shed so many tears at one luncheon. We didn't know that a contact could slide to the end of a person's nose and stay in that position until removed with a napkin. Gertie's new frames are very attractive. ❀

Dear Maggie Montclair,

I had the good fortune to be married to two wonderful men. Each man is the father of two of my four children. I have decided to plan my funeral, but I have a problem of where to be buried. My children have agreed that I should be cremated with half my ashes buried with each man.

Our problem arises with this question: can I have my name and date of birth and death inscribed on both monuments? They will be in different towns.

Ashes in Two Towns in Texas

Dear Ashes in Two Towns,

You and your children have come up with a great solution. I hope it is legal in Texas. Call a lawyer and make sure you can arrange this. *M*

P.S.: Gertie was married four times and has made and paid for her funeral arrangements. The only information she will share is the name of the mortuary. She says that on the day of her demise, her children will need a good laugh. ❀

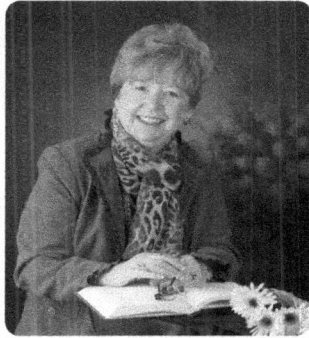

About the Author

For decades, Janet Laird shared her morning coffee with Ann Landers, Erma Bombeck, and Heloise. Now, writing as Maggie Montclair—her readers call Maggie the Ann Landers for widows—Janet shares the survival techniques that she and her friends have used to move forward after the loss of their husbands.

Janet was born and raised in Oelwein, Iowa, and is a graduate of Upper Iowa University. A widow for twenty-two years, she currently lives in Omaha. She travels as often as possible with her Red Hat Chapter, "The Dingbats in Red Hats."

There are as many approaches to widowhood as there are widows. Like daisies, Janet hopes you will pick and choose which gems of advice ring true for you.

Janet agrees with this advice from Maggie Montclair, "Don't be afraid to stretch yourself and get out of your comfort zone. If you haven't made a few mistakes, you either haven't traveled very far or you have stayed in the 'safety zone' and led an unfulfilling life."

Acknowledgments

$\mathcal{T}$ hanks to my favorite aunt and dear friend Lois G. Harvey, a talented poet, who has allowed me to share some of her lovely poetic words.

And to my widowed friends who, over the past two decades, have shared their trials and successes with me. These are your stories. Any one of you could have written this little book.

Also thank you to my daughter, Nicole, and son Joel and wife Carol, and son Michael and wife Duana for all the love and support they give me. I love you dearly.

Without Concierge Marketing, Inc., this little book would still be rattling around in my head. I can't thank you enough. You made my dream come true.

God bless you all.

Quick Guide
to Maggie's Answers to
These Important Questions

I know you are not supposed to make big decisions for at least a year, but … [chapter 1]

People say, "Call me if there is anything I can do for you." [chapter 1]

How much longer before my life is normal again? [chapter 1]

It has been a year, and I just can't move on. [chapter 1]

I know this must sound terrible, but I smiled all the way home from the cemetery. [chapter 1]

I still dread eating alone. [chapter 2]

I have season tickets to the symphony, but my friends either go with their husbands or won't leave their husbands to go out for an evening. [chapter 2]

When my husband died, I was left to grieve and care for our mentally challenged son who had grown into adulthood. [chapter 2]

I am afraid to be alone at night. [chapter 2]

I thought our adult daughter and I would be able to live together and even enjoy many activities. [chapter 2]

My children are insisting that I move. But I want to stay in my home. [chapter 3]

I have joined a widows' group that has many social activities, but it seems there is some unspoken rule that I don't know about. [chapter 3]

The husband of one of our friends called and asked me to lunch. [chapter 3]

I am having trouble making new friends. [chapter 3]

What is wrong with me? Why are my former friends ignoring me? [chapter 3]

I have a wonderful, well-educated, beautiful daughter who says I embarrass her. [chapter 4]

I need serious surgery. [chapter 4]

Believe it or not, I'm still raising children—my grandchildren. [chapter 4]

My son is worried about my safety. [chapter 4]

My friends and I were having lunch last week when the subject of those alert buttons you wear around your neck or wrist came up. [chapter 4]

I can't believe that my grandchildren have become so rude and greedy. [chapter 4]

I just got home from the funeral of a dear friend. It was so sad and upsetting to see her children arguing with each other. [chapter 4]

I'm just wondering, what can I leave my children and my grandchildren that was a part of my life that they will want to keep as a way to remember me? [chapter 4]

My widowed sister moved in with me, and I have discovered she is a hoarder. How can I save my home and my sanity? [chapter 4]

I have been dating the most wonderful man. … Are these so-called red flags really important, or can I tell my daughter to quit worrying and let me be happy? [chapter 5]

I have been widowed for almost ten years. He thinks we should each retire and live in my house. [chapter 5]

I have met the most wonderful man, but my friends and family don't like him. [chapter 5]

My daughter is upset with me because I have started dating. [chapter 5]

I want to meet a man to spend time with. I am tempted to check out Internet dating. [chapter 5]

My doctor told me to get a treadmill and walk thirty minutes every day. I bought the treadmill, and my son-in-law set it up. That was the easy part. [chapter 6]

I have adjusted to widowhood and have a happy and full life. There is one thing I would like to do, but it seems a foolish waste of money. [chapter 6]

My problem is that my new friends and I go out to lunch so much that I have gained much more weight than I should. [chapter 6]

Why won't clothing manufacturers design beautiful clothes for older women? [chapter 6]

Last week while I was getting my hair done,
I glanced in the mirror and saw my mother.
[chapter 6]

Am I dreaming, or can I really look and feel
attractive again? [chapter 6]

I had the good fortune to be married to two
wonderful men. Each man is the father of two
of my four children. I have decided to plan my
funeral, but I have a problem of where to be
buried. [chapter 6]

Quotes from "Mama Said..." *by Lois G. Harvey*

"Don't try to do everything right now.
Save some things to do when you are older."

❀ ❀ ❀

"At least one day a year
every working person should
call in sick, not make the bed,
schlepp around in an old robe,
eat what he pleases, rest,
read something comforting,
and let the world
take care of itself."

❀ ❀ ❀

"If you don't want to
do something, just say:
'Sorry, I can't do that.'
Make no excuses."

❀ ❀ ❀

"I hear better with my glasses on."

❀ ❀ ❀

"Busy mothers should
use the help they have —
their children.
It's good training
and good sense."

❀ ❀ ❀

"Discipline your children
before they are four.
They won't remember,
and will love you more."

❀ ❀ ❀

"On your husband's birthday
send a 'Thank You' card
to your mother-in-law."

❀ ❀ ❀

" 'Tis a lucky person
who, in one lifetime knows
one poet
one lover
and one friend."

❁   ❁   ❁

"Help your grandma;
you'll be old someday, too."

❁   ❁   ❁

www.ingramcontent.com/pod-product-compliance
Lightning Source LLC
LaVergne TN
LVHW011242080426
835509LV00005B/605